Also by Mardie Caldwell

AdoptingOnline.com

Adoption: Your Step-by-Step Guide

The Healthcare Professional's Adoption Guide

So I Was Thinking About Adoption...

Considering Your Choices

Mardie Caldwell, C.O.A.P.

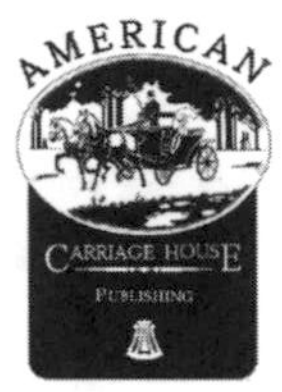

American Carriage House Publishing

So I Was Thinking About Adoption . . .

Considering Your Choices

Published by American Carriage House Publishing

P.O. Box 1130 Nevada City, CA 95959

Library of Congress Control Number: 2008934158

Caldwell, Mardie.

ISBN 978-0-9705734-5-2 (softcover)

Printed and bound in the United States of America

This book is dedicated to my son's first mother, Donna, his beautiful birth mother.

Today is our son's 16th birthday. Tears fill my eyes, as I remember many years ago, how she chose adoption because of her deep love and selfless concern for her son's best future.

God bless you across the miles!

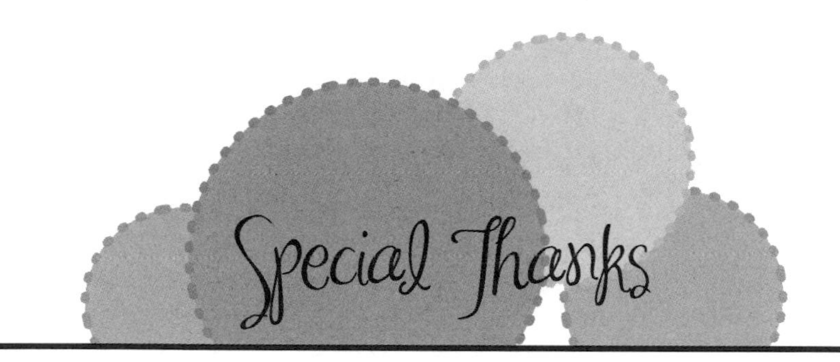

I want to thank the following contributors to this book: Heidi Zimmerman, Heather Featherston, Briana Caldwell, and Amie Weaver, who worked long hours to make this book what it is today. Rebekah Tennis, for designing a wonderful cover and interior for the book. Thanks to Darlene Breed for editing the first drafts of this labor of love. A very special thanks goes to all of my hardworking staff, who have been so terrific in their support and assistance with this book.

Table of Contents

CHAPTER ONE:

So I was thinking about Adoption...

I got pregnant when I was only 15...I was terrified to tell my mom, but then the day came when I couldn't zip up my pants any more and she found out!

Instead of going to school, she drove me to the doctor, with tears in our eyes. Turns out, I was already 5 months pregnant; guess that made sense, the baby was already kicking me all the time.

The thought of being a mother was a far-away idea. As my belly got bigger and my due date came closer, reality started to sink in.

I didn't have baby things or the money to buy them. I didn't have a job, heck I hadn't even finished high school. I think that is when I really started to consider my choices... so, I was thinking about adoption...

Megan

Let's be honest, women don't plan on choosing adoption for their children. You aren't reading this book because you want to be a "birth mother." You need help and want information. You need to learn more about the choices you have with adoption.

Right answers...Right reasons

Your head may be spinning from your family and friends telling you what they think you should do. Parents tell you one thing. Friends tell you something else. Once you have the facts, you'll feel much more in control, and ready to make the right choices for the right reasons.

Before we start, let's get rid of some old, guilt-trip sayings or "big ideas." They're old-fashioned, hurtful, and just plain untrue - and they go something like this:

- *She doesn't care or she wouldn't give her baby away.*
- *Adoption is a big secret and she doesn't know what's going on.*
- *She'll never forgive herself if she gives her baby away.*
- *If she's old enough to get pregnant, she's old enough to be a parent.*

These comments are NOT true, and people who say these things don't know about adoption today. Today, we know that for many women, placing their babies and children for adoption is a smart and caring way to provide a lifetime of love and stability in a rock-solid family.

Please read this guide all the way through before you make any decision. If you understand the truth, and listen to what's going on in your heart and head, you will have greater peace about the choices you make. You will also have confidence that you are making the right decision for you and your baby for all the *right* reasons.

Why do women choose adoption?

Babies are hard work. You've got to feed, change, bathe, amuse, protect, and clean up after them. It's a big, 24/7 responsibility. As a mom, you've got to be ready to put your life and outside interests on hold to focus on your child. Your baby needs time and attention twenty-four hours a day. But what if you're not ready to give up your life?

There are many reasons women choose adoption, such as:

- *Not ready to be a mom*
- *Situations that prevent parenting, such as mental illness or jail sentence*
- *No support from baby's father*
- *Desire for a solid, two-parent family*
- *Safety and stability*
- *College plans*
- *Opportunity for a solid future*
- *Prior involvement with Child Protective Services*
- *Cannot afford another child*
- *Lifestyle*
- *Rape*

Whatever your reason for considering adoption today, you are not alone. And the good news is that women choosing adoption can play an active role in just about every step of the process. You can choose the parents for your child, receive counseling, create your own adoption plan, and meet the adoptive parents. You can even receive help with pregnancy, living and medical costs, if your state allows it.

What kind of a parent would I be?

It's totally normal to consider what kind of parent you would be. Choosing your child's parents through adoption lets you evaluate what kind of parents they will be. But what about you? What kind of parent are you ready to be?

- *Are you truly able to provide for yourself and your baby on your own?*
- *Is the father of your baby likely to help you money-wise and emotionally? If not, will you be able to cope by yourself?*
- *Do you have school or work that will take up a lot of your time?*
- *Have family and friends offered to help you care for your child?*
- *Do they always do what they say they will?*
- *Can you afford to feed, clothe, educate, and get medical attention for your child?*
- *Can you give your child the kind of life he or she deserves? The kind of life you want for them?*
- *Are you truly ready to give up your life to become mom to your baby?*

It takes courage to be honest with yourself. Your answers will help you focus on what you want for your baby.

A Lifetime Plan for My Child

List what you can offer your child if you were to parent him/her:

1. Love
2.
3.
4.
5.
6.
7.
8.
9.
10.

How do I know adoption is a good choice for my baby?

If you are not ready to be a parent or you are not able to take responsibility for the growth and development of your child, you can still give your baby the gift of life by choosing adoption. You can choose the way your baby will be raised by selecting a stable, loving family for him. You can even choose a family that has interests you desire, like religious beliefs or hobbies.

At birth, you can see your baby, hold him, and even name him if you wish. As your child grows, you can receive letters, photos, and even visits, allowing you to watch him grow up strong and happy, surrounded by the warmth of a loving family. You can always be a part of your child's life. You can reach for your own goals, knowing that your child is cared for in every way.

Adoption may not be right for everyone. You need to evaluate what you are prepared to provide and determine if that is enough for your baby.

Is it selfish to consider adoption? Is it selfish to consider parenting?

No. Neither decision is selfish if you are making it based on the right reasons.

Adoption can be one of the most unselfish decisions you can make. It gives your child the opportunity to have a family who has the time, resources, and

A Lifetime Plan for My Child

List what an adoptive family can offer your child through an open adoption:

1. Love
2. Stable home-life
3. Financial security
4. Emotionally ready & willing to parent
5. One or two parent home
6. Ability to provide sports, hobbies, music, etc.
7. Welcoming grandparents & other relatives
8. Quality medical, dental, eye care, and education
9. Vacations, opportunity to travel
10. Stay-at-home mom (optional)
11. Knowledge that his/her birth parents cared enough to choose the best for their child's life

Are You Ready to be a Parent?

1) Do you have the financial resources to care for this child?
2) Do you have the help you need to raise your child?
3) Will those who are offering to help be there long-term?
4) Will the child have two committed parents?
5) How are you feeling emotionally about being a parent?
6) What do you want for your child's life?
7) What do you want for your life?
8) Are you and the father willing to sacrifice your lifestyle to be good parents?
9) What kind of childhood did you **want** as a child? Can you provide that for **your** child?
10) Why do you want to be a parent?
11) Will being a mother make you a better person?
12) Do you feel that having a child will give you someone to love? Someone to love you in return?
13) Do you think parenting will keep you and the father together?
14) Do you know someone who has been in a similar situation? What are the choices they made? How is their life now?

ability to cherish this baby *just as you may want to do*. It is hard to admit that you may not be able to be a mom right now; however the good news is that adoption is not goodbye forever. You can choose to remain involved in your child's life, and your child will know why you chose another path for them.

Parenting a child is difficult. Love is not enough to provide what a child needs to thrive. Even in a committed relationship or with the help of family and friends, being a parent is a full time job!

What is the difference between closed, open, and semi-open adoption?

In a closed adoption, you let your adoption professional choose the adoptive family for you. After the adoption, you will have no contact with the family or with the child.

In semi-open adoption, only your first names are shared with the adoptive parents. You may have some say in the selection of adoptive parents, followed by little or no contact with the child or family.

In an open adoption, you may choose your child's family. You may also stay in touch. Some women want letters and photos, and others want occasional visits and phone calls.

Your baby benefits from open adoption in the following ways:

- *Your child will come to know that you loved him enough to want the very best for him.*
- *Your child will know why you chose adoption for him.*
- *Your child will have the opportunity to receive information about his biological family.*
- *Your child will have the chance to know his genealogy and medical information.*
- *Your child will have the opportunity for ongoing communication with his birth parents.*

What is the difference between adoption and foster care?

"Wow! I know adoption was the right choice. It scares me to think I almost missed the opportunity to give my child and this family a forever gift."

-Heidi in Maine

Adoption gives you the opportunity to choose the life you want for your child. It is permanent, although you can choose to remain a part of your child's life. Right now, you have choices and control.

Foster care may be a short-term or temporary arrangement and it may or may not allow you any choices regarding where your child will go. Most children placed in foster care in the U.S. are there because of neglect, abuse, or abandonment. Once a child is in the foster care system, it can be very difficult to get them back out.

If your child is currently in *voluntary* foster care, your adoption coordinator will work with you and an attorney to determine the steps to be taken to have your child legally adopted into a permanent home at no cost to you. Options may be available to help you choose what happens with your child's future if you take just one step. Contact the National Adoption Hotline at 1-800-923-6602 to get the help you need.

The father of your baby

The father of your baby is usually referred to as the "birth father" in adoption language. Whether or not you are involved with him, parenting this child is his responsibility just as much as yours. If you decide to parent, he will have the obligation to pay child support, and the opportunity to share custody.

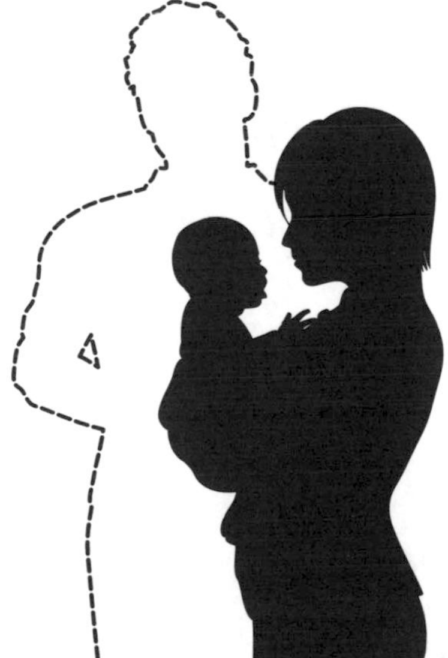

Ask yourself a few questions about your baby's father.

- *Is he someone you would want to grow old with?*
- *Will he be a good role model for your child?*
- *Is he responsible? Does he have a job?*
- *Does he pay his own way?*
- *Does he party, drink too much, or do drugs?*
- *Has he been faithful to you?*
- *Does he have other kids? What kind of father is he to them?*
- *Do your family and friends like him?*
- *Has he been in jail?*
- *Are you putting your safety at risk by parenting this child?*
- *Would you want your child to grow up and marry a man just like this guy? Or, if your baby is a boy, would you want him to grow up and be just like him?*
- *Is he kind towards his parents?*
- *Does he have a history of verbal, physical, or sexual abuse?*
- *Does he follow through on what he says he will do?*

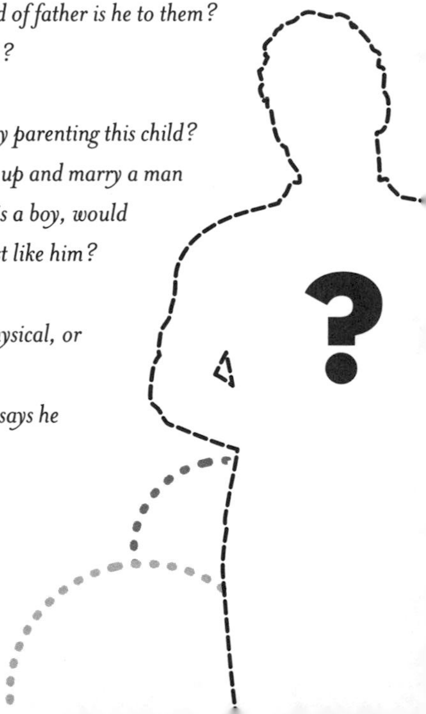

I've been dating the father of my baby. Wouldn't it be better if we just got married and tried to raise the child together?

Perhaps, as long as you are not marrying simply because of the pregnancy. Marriage for the wrong reason has a greater chance of failure, compared to a relationship that has had time to develop without the pressure of an unplanned pregnancy. Be honest with yourself about your relationship with your baby's father. The decision to marry should be because you are both committed to each other and want to marry, not because you are having a baby together.

Think about what you want for your life before adding marriage and parenting. Don't put your child's future at risk if you and the father

Anna's Story

Anna knew she had to make a decision about her pregnancy, and soon. She was running out of time.

Her mother said she should place the baby in a family with a mom and dad. Her boy-friend said he would pay to terminate the pregnancy. Her best friend said she should keep the baby. Her head was spinning. She didn't know what to do.

She decided to call a counselor. After a few hard, but caring talks, Anna was able to make a choice that was right for her and her situation. She wanted to move to another city until the baby was born, then place the baby with adoptive parents she had selected herself. Her boyfriend was relieved, and her best friend was upset for awhile, but got over it.

Today, Anna reflects, "Talking with some-one else let me escape from the pressure I was under. I was able to honestly consider my baby's future, and mine too! When I met the family I had selected as "ideal," I felt they truly respected me. By doing what I thought was best, I could be proud of my decision. Ultimately, I did the most loving thing possible; I created a beautiful life for the child I created."

are not ready to give your full attention to being parents. It's okay to not be ready or to decide that you want more out of life before "settling down."

Consider what kind of home life you want for your child. Are you ready and able to provide a stable and safe home? Is your man? If not, adoption can offer the home life you desire for your child.

Your parents: The birth grandparents

Some birth grandparents are supportive and involved in the adoption plan. In fact, some even make the first phone calls to an adoption professional to get help for their child. Others don't understand adoption and may even try to change your mind.

It's important to know that even if you are very young, birth grandparents typically have no rights in adoption by law. They can't force you to parent your baby or to choose adoption, no matter how young you are. They can definitely make it difficult and pressure you, but remember it is *your* decision. Many women have created a written adoption or parenting plan to present to their parents in difficult family situations.

CHAPTER TWO: Writing it all down...

Journaling

A great way to help with considering all of your choices is to write your thoughts and emotions down. Adding pen to paper can be a very personal and reflective journey. Taking the time to reflect on your feelings about your pregnancy and your unborn child can be a helpful process. Perhaps you want to write a letter to your baby or to yourself sharing the reasons behind your decisions. This may seem difficult, but you may find it makes the healing a little easier.

Kassie's Journal

March – Today is the day, I never expected. Not now, not this way. I am staring at the pregnancy test, the one I took three times last week. But today, you were confirmed. The doctor says you are healthy. How can he know, you haven't even been alive for a month, but still something inside me feels you are here for a reason. I have thought about getting rid of you. I don't think I have it in me. I don't know where we will go from here, but I hope it works out. I am scared and a little lonely, but something about you brings me comfort.

April – I talked with your father today. He doesn't want you. I think he would love you, how could anybody not love you. But he won't pick up the phone anymore. He says he will pay for me to get rid of you. I told him I can't. My family doesn't know about you yet, I am waiting to tell them. You have two brothers and a sister. They don't know either. I started thinking about a name for you, but then I stopped. I am afraid I will not be the parent you should have.

May – I love you. You are getting bigger, I am gaining weight. I can't afford rent this month. I am not sure how I will take care of you. My friends say they would keep you. I wish your father would have stayed around; it would have been easier then. I am starting to cry a lot. My family is worried about me. I don't talk much about you. I am starting to doubt my decisions. I want you to know I want the best for you.

June – I called an adoption place today. I talked to them for a long time. They are sending me families to look at. I am confused and sad, but maybe there is a reason for it all. You are starting to move around. I talked to my family today. They think that adoption might be a good idea. I guess they are supportive. I still wish there was something I could do to make it work out. Maybe I will buy a lottery ticket.

July – I was nervous about talking to the adoptive family today. I want them to like you. They seem nice and their pictures are really cute. I can write you as often as I want and even see you. They live in the country with a big house. You would have a sister. All I want for you is to be happy and grow up loved. I started writing you a letter today to tell you how I feel. I will miss you.

August – I talked with another woman today who placed her baby for adoption four years ago. She said the first year is the hardest. She said she knows her baby is healthy and happy and she gets pictures all the time. She told me to keep loving you, even when it hurts. I think that was good advice. She said I will cry a lot and I will miss you, but she also said that healing takes time, and that you will have a beautiful life. I feel a little better.

September – I talked with your dad today. He knows about the adoption plan, he doesn't want to know about the family, but he said he will sign the papers. I wish you could have known him a little bit, but I hope you don't grow up like him. Your adoptive family called again. They are sending a baby blanket for when I deliver. Sometimes I get really confused about everything. I wonder about the life I could give you, and I wonder about watching you grow up. I wish I could make it work, but I know I can't give you what you need. Sometimes I wish I could make everything go away.

October – Today was a good day. You kicked a lot. I met the adoptive family. We went to the park. It was beautiful, and they are really nice. We talked a lot about your name. I think you will like them. They brought pictures of their pets and I met your sister. She is five. She talked to you and pressed her little hand on my stomach. She said she loved you. I hope you could hear her. The adoptive family will be there at the hospital. I am getting a little nervous and a little excited.

November – I am ready to be done now. There are still a lot of emotions going on. The hardest thing is dealing with my family. They think I don't love you, but that's not true. I love you very much. I want you to have everything that I can't give you. I wish you were old enough to understand. This is the hardest thing I have ever done. I hope that one day you will learn that this was the most unselfish decision I have ever made.

December – I delivered you today. You are beautiful. Somehow I thought it would be different with the adoptive family there. They love you already. I love you still. I watched you smile and wondered if you will look like that ten years from now. I got to hold you and say my goodbyes and I stayed up to watch you sleep. There is a lot I wish I could say, but somehow words don't seem to be enough. They will make a good family, and you will be a good daughter, and I hope when I see you, you will remember me. I am keeping your baby footprints and your ID bracelet and even though it hurts, I know in my heart that this is the right choice.

My Journal

My Journal

My Journal

CHAPTER THREE:
I have a few questions...

Here are some real answers to questions you may have about how adoption works. At any time you can speak to a caring professional by calling National Adoption Hotline at 1-800-923-6602.

1. Are there any costs to me?

No, you will not need to pay for anything. Adoptive parents pay for legal fees, medical bills not covered by insurance, and counseling fees. The family may also be able to provide assistance with pregnancy related expenses to help you, which can include rent and food, depending on state laws. You also can receive help with some of your needs such as maternity clothes, household items, and other necessities from places like **www.BirthmotherBlessings.com.**

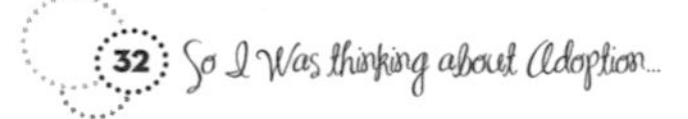

2. Will I have any say in who will adopt my child?

Yes. In an open adoption, you have all kinds of choices. You can be actively involved in the adoption for your child. You can choose the adoptive parents and even meet them in person. In fact, you'll find that the closer you get to the placement, the more you may want a face-to-face meeting. After all, these will be the people who will be raising your child. You'll want to know as much as you can about them and that you've made the right decision. You can ask your adoption professional to mail you information about adoptive families or view them online at **www.LifetimeAdoption.com.**

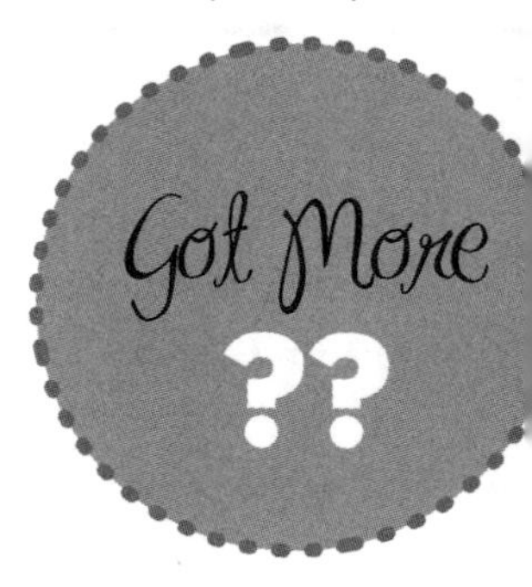

3. How can I be sure that the family I choose for my baby are good people?

Your adoption professional will screen and pre-qualify all the adoptive families that are working with them. A licensed social worker will do a detailed home study evaluation and visit the adoptive family's home. This home study evaluation includes a background check, medical and financial evaluations, and FBI screening. You can be assured that your baby will be raised within a loving and safe family environment. If you wish, you can speak personally to families and decide whom you feel you want to adopt and raise your child.

4. How much will my child know about me?

It is entirely up to you to decide what type of contact you want with the adoptive family and your child. In an open adoption, you and your child's adoptive family can have some contact throughout the years. This can vary from letters and photos to visits once or twice a year. You may wish to write a letter or send photos to your child or children, letting them know how you made this decision out of your love for them. This letter can be given to your child when he or she is old enough to understand. It is important that the adoptive family have access to your medical records/history for your child's medical reference in the future. You can pass on any information about yourself and your life to your child's adoptive parents. Your child will know that this decision was made in order to give them the best future possible.

For Answers Call
1 (800) 923-6602
National Adoption Hotline

5. What if my child is older, can I make an adoption plan?

There are loving families seeking children of all ages and races. Your adoption professional will work hard to find just the right family for you to consider for the adoption. You will be able to decide on the type of contact you wish to have after the adoption.

6. What if my child has a disability or medical problem? Are there adoptive families available?

Yes, there are adoptive families that are prepared and willing to provide a loving and supportive home for a child with special needs. There is a loving and safe home for every child.
Just call the National Adoption Hotline at 1-800-923-6602 and receive details on how to get started.

7. What if I go into labor and have not made an adoption plan?

You can call an adoption professional directly from the hospital. They can have a family available within hours. In most states, the adoptive family will be able to take the baby home from the hospital; this will allow your baby to start bonding with their adoptive family right away.

If you are concerned about Child Protective Services, it is important that you know you have the right to make an adoption plan for your child. You have the choice to decide the type of home you would like your child to grow up in, instead of the foster care system. There are adoption professionals open for emergencies on all weekends, holidays, and throughout the night, call 1-800-923-6602 anytime, 24/7 for help.

8. What if I change my mind and decide I want to raise my child myself?

Before all forms are signed, you may change your mind. It's recommended that you make this decision sooner than later since the longer you wait, the harder it will be. For now, go slowly and take things one step at a time.

If you want counseling, be sure to request it. Remember there is no cost to you. Counseling may help you clarify your feelings and just because you feel sorrow or guilt, it does not mean that your decision to move forward with adoption was incorrect. This is a good time to evaluate if your living situation has changed. What were the reasons you chose adoption in the first place?

9. Does the father of my baby have any say in the adoption?

His rights are similar to yours and vary by state. If the two of you disagree about adoption, or if you are no longer together, your adoption professional will work with an attorney to determine if his rights can be terminated. For legal reasons, he will most likely have to be contacted, but you don't have to be the one to do it. If you don't want to speak to him, share your concerns with your adoption professional.

It is always easier for you if the child's father signs a waiver and provides his medical information. If he is not willing or is not around to do this, an adoption plan is possible without his participation. However, if he is known, he must be notified of the adoption. The attorney working for you will advise the father of your decision and let him know of his options.

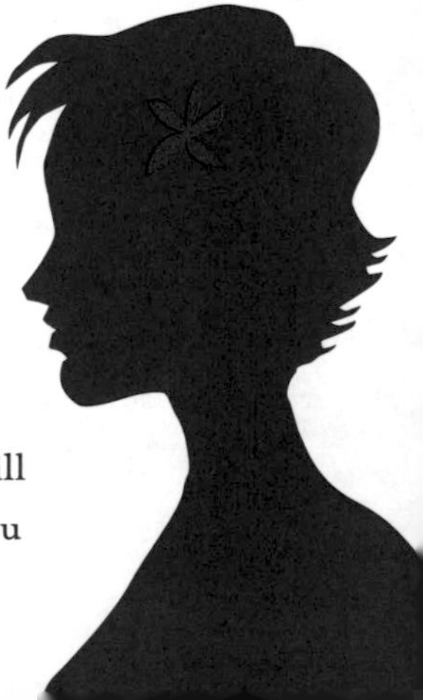

10. I am a single parent and facing a prison sentence. Can I find adoptive parents for my baby or older children?

Yes. An adoption professional can work with you in finding a loving adoptive family that will legally adopt your children. It is important you realize that adoption is permanent and legally binding. Adoption is not foster care or temporary care.

You may wish to seek out any family member that you feel could provide a stable and loving home for your children if possible. If you have attempted to do this and feel that you prefer for an adoption professional to find a suitable home for your child, then they will be happy to assist you.

11. I am homeless and pregnant. Is there a home for mothers or a place for me to go?

Yes, services and assistance may be available to you. Depending on your age, you will have a variety of support services such as relocation to another town, sharing a home with another birth mother, maternity care homes and studio apartments. Your adoption coordinator can help you find housing, and they sometimes have families that are interested in housing a birth mother for the term of her pregnancy. Some women want to move to another area until after the baby is born and others want to stay in their own town. Much will be determined by how far along you are in your pregnancy, what your situation is, and your plans for your child.

If needed, they will refer you to other services, answer your questions and provide useful information to help you decide what your options are. If you are in this situation, it is best to call the National Adoption Hotline as soon as you can at 1-800-923-6602, so it can be decided what your needs are and get help for you quickly.

12. I need help paying my medical bills and my rent. Can the adoptive parents help me with this?

In most states, adoptive parents are allowed to help with pregnancy-related expenses, such as living, medical, and travel expenses. If you have state or private medical insurance, the adoptive parents may be able to pay any portions unpaid by insurance, such as co-payments. Living expenses may include rent, utilities, and maternity clothing. Travel may include transportation to and from your doctor's office. In most states, living expenses may be paid up to six weeks after the birth. Payment of living expenses can only begin after you have filled out the required forms, selected the adoptive parents, and have both agreed to go forward with an adoption plan.

Please let your adoption professional know as soon as possible what your needs are. You can also visit the resources section at the back of this book for additional help.

13. Are there families of other races to adopt my baby?

Yes! You may view waiting adoptive families of many races by visiting:

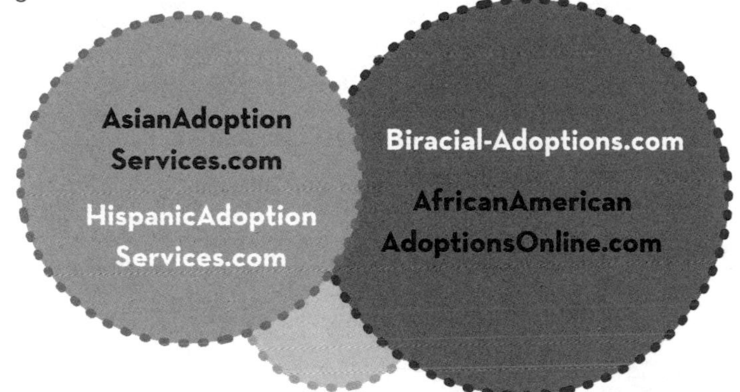

You can read about the lifestyle of these families and view their photos before speaking to them on the phone. Many families may not be racially diverse themselves, but are open and willing to provide a loving and supportive home for a child of any race.

You may have even more questions than are answered here; remember there is no such thing as a silly question. If you do, please know you can call and speak with someone 24 hours a day at the National Adoption Hotline, 1-800-923-6602.

Questions to ask

CHAPTER FOUR:

Spilling the beans...

So this idea of telling the people closest to you about adoption might seem a little scary. You don't have to tell anyone if you don't want to, because all of the services offered to you are confidential. This decision is up to you; however, it may be easier in the long run if everyone is up-front and honest with each other. The best way to do this is to choose a time when you feel you have their attention and some privacy. This means being honest with yourself first and then being honest with your friends, family and the father of your child.

Your friends...

In theory, true friends are supposed to be with you for the long haul. That means that if you decide to tell them about your pregnancy then they will be supportive of whatever decision you decide is best for you and your baby. They may have different reactions at first, so be prepared. They might try and judge you or make you change your mind.

Remember, friends often want to be helpful and they may tell you that they will support you or even help take care of the baby. The truth is that babies take a lot of work, and while your friends might be willing to help you in a crunch, in the long term they won't be able to provide the kind of support you need. Keep your good friends close and ask them to help you through the hard times. They can be good support for doctor's appointments or to go to counseling, or even to help you break the news to family, that you are considering adoption.

Your parents...

If you are looking for some advice on how to tell your parents, the best approach is to be mature. Tell them that you need to talk to them about a serious matter and ask them to be respectful and not to interrupt you until you have finished. Explain to them what is going on and ask for their support, understanding and help.

This news is likely shocking to your parents, so have a little understanding and patience with them, and realize that they might get angry, but handling the conversation with maturity will make a huge difference. It's best if you can avoid arguing, even though it might be hard, especially if you feel judged. Give them some time and space to digest the information then approach them again with a plan about how you intend on handling the situation.

Wendy Shares her Plans

Wendy was 23, living at home with her parents and her 3-year-old son. When she found out she was pregnant, she was fearful of what her parents' reaction would be. She called me and we spoke on the phone. We developed a plan just for her. I gave her suggestions on how to talk to her parents, to pick the best time, along with the details to prove she had been responsible enough to think it all out.

Wendy was sure of her decision about adoption. She decided to focus her time and energy on her son and to continue working. I also offered to speak to her parents and to be a support to her the night she told them.

Wendy's parents were disappointed, but not surprised, as Wendy had begun to show. When Wendy shared their reaction, she said it went better than expected, with her plans in hand and her thoughts in front of her. She was able to explain to them how open adoption works, and how she had thought through all of her options. She was able to give intelligent answers to their questions.

Narrowing the choices down to two adoptive families' profiles she thought were perfect, she knew exactly what to show her parents.

The birth father hadn't wanted anything to do with her once he found out she was pregnant. In fact, he had told her to get an abortion. Wendy had already had one abortion and had no intention of having another.

She asked for help with her expenses from her adoptive family for the last month of her pregnancy, and the adoptive parents agreed.

She continued to work as a store clerk throughout her entire pregnancy, delivered her baby, and then went back to work and to night school. She receives yearly photos and updates about her daughter. She admits that her adoption plan was hard to put down on paper because it made it real to her, but it also helped her in realizing that it was the best thing she could do for her baby and her son.

"When my daughter was born, I just looked at her," Wendy said. "I studied her fingers and toes and kissed the top of her head. I told her how much I loved her and how wonderful her life would be with two people that loved her as much as I did."

"Then," she continued, "I knew I had done the right thing. The adoptive parents came in and carried her home as we had planned, and although I cried for the next three days, I never had a doubt that what I did wasn't the best for her and us. I have learned a lot since my adoption and I know the choice I made was one I thought out and planned. I have no regrets."

Baby's father...

When thinking about talking with the father, there are a couple of things to think about and consider:

- *Do you feel he will be supportive?*
- *Do you think he will stick with you for the long haul?*
- *Do you think he will eventually marry you?*
- *What are his goals and dreams?*
- *Do they align with yours?*
- *Is he willing to support you in telling your parents?*
- *Is he willing to take responsibility for his actions?*
- *Has he considered what you want for your life?*
- *Has he been responsible for his decisions?*
- *How do his parents feel?*
- *Does he have other children?*

It is important to evaluate your relationship with real honesty here. If you aren't still together or if you are afraid of him, you want to make sure your safety is the first priority. Consider the following questions:

- *What do you think his reaction will be once he finds out you're pregnant?*
- *Do you want him involved in your life – for at least the next 18 years?*
- *Is he willing or able to pay child support?*
- *Is he the type of father you want for your children?*
- *If he is violent, have you called the police?*
- *Does he have a criminal history?*

It is important that you take all of these things into consideration, for your safety and the well-being of your child.

Planning ahead...

Before you have any of these conversations, these are important issues to consider:

- *How will you provide for the child financially?*
- *Where will you live?*
- *Do you have help?*
- *Are you and the father still together?*
- *Does he work or is he willing to start?*
- *Are you planning on getting married?*
- *What are your plans for finishing school?*
- *Make a list of your goals for the next two years–how will the child fit into these?*
- *What are your expectations from your parents?*
- *If your parents provide support for you,*
    - *Are you willing to listen to their rules?*
    - *Are you willing to let them help you decide how to parent?*
- *Is making an adoption plan something you are willing to consider?*

If the answer to the last question is yes, then let's move ahead. Do you feel comfortable sharing your decision with your family, friends, and the father? Where do you find the most support? Making an adoption plan is a personal decision, but it can really help to have those you trust there to support you in your plans.

For example, you can share the profiles of the adoptive families you like with them, so that your family can see the loving families you have chosen. You can also have them help you write a letter to your child, or ask them to come with you when you meet the family, if you like. You can have anyone you like with you at the hospital to help you through the birth. It is important that you take the time to honor your feelings and your needs during your pregnancy and being honest with those closest to you can help you make this journey a little easier.

How to Tell Your Kids About Your Adoption Plan

If you have kids, they may wonder about your pregnancy and adoption decision. Depending on their age, you can tell them that you are going to have a baby, but won't be able to take care of the baby. Babies need lots of attention, and you may not be able to care for any more children right now. You might explain that you don't have a crib, special baby food, or a stroller to push the baby in, and there wouldn't be anyone to care for the baby while you are at work.

Tell them that you have found a family who want a baby to love, and that they are going to take care of the baby in your tummy. Your child might be worried that the other family will adopt them too, so it's a good idea to explain that they will still live with you. They will always be that baby's sister or brother, but the baby just won't live with you.

You know your kids, and you know what they will be able to handle and understand. Many women have chosen not to tell their kids who are very young because it is too complicated for the child and too difficult for themselves. You may wish to discuss this with a trusted friend or relative who knows your child.

For more information, here is a children's book you might share with your child that explains adoption:

Sam's Sister *by Juliet C. Bond*

My goals for the future

CHAPTER FIVE:

The real deal about parenting & adoption...

Sure, parenting starts out with a cute cuddly baby that is going to love you and look to you for guidance and protection. But there is a lot more to parenting than that.

Being a parent is a full time job, with a lot of responsibility. It is important that you think about how being a parent may change your lifestyle permanently.

Right now you may be thinking how hard it will be to place your child with an adoptive family. And you are right. Making an adoption plan is never an easy decision, but if you are thinking about the best long term decision for your child, adoption can be the most loving gift you can give.

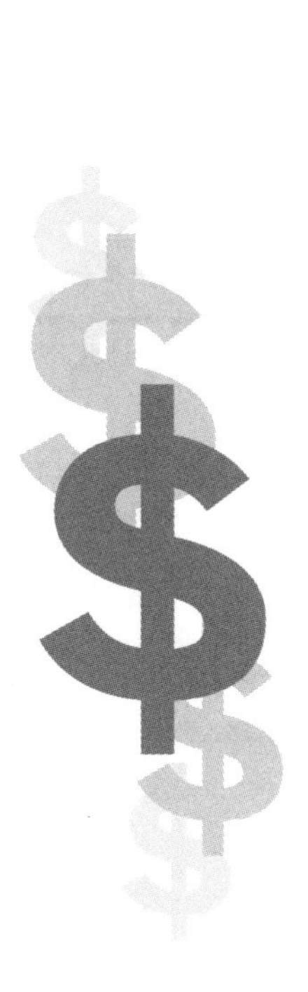

COST OF RAISING A CHILD FROM BIRTH TO AGE 18:

Single Parent	2 Parents
$122,590	$130,800

$46,000 in housing
$27,000 in food
$16,000 in transportation
$9,000 in clothing
$7,000 in healthcare
$9,000 in childcare and education
$10,000 miscellaneous expenses

**And this is just the bare minimum. This does not include any special gifts, or if your child gets very ill, or the cost of any additional education, like if you want your child to go to college.*

"I really love my baby and have struggled with adoption, but I don't want to bring my baby up in poverty."

- Becky in Washington

"I could raise my daughter, but she would be in childcare all day while I worked. I just don't want that for her..."

-Marie in California

A Life Changing Decision

My story is probably similar to many of you. I am a 20 year old woman, who thought she had it all together. Well, actually not all of it, but enough to parent my first daughter. I am not going to lie; having her has been the hardest and most wonderful journey of my life. When I got pregnant the first time, I figured that it would be difficult, but somehow we would make it work. I thought that the baby's father would eventually learn to love me, but he took off, and that left me alone to raise my daughter. Without the help of my parents, I don't think I would have made it this far.

At first she was so cute. She would snuggle with me and we would cry together, and eventually my body healed, and I was actually making it work. My parents watched her in the morning while I went to school and then I would get home and take over. It wasn't much harder than a new puppy at first. I would show her to all my friends and we would talk bad about her dad, and somehow it made me feel a little better. But then she got bigger and I couldn't carry her everywhere. And she kept growing out of her clothes, needed more food, and pretty soon all of the extra cash I had saved was gone.

When she turned two my parents asked me to move out. Move out? What do you mean move out? I just graduated in June from high school, what kind of job am I supposed to get? It is now October, and I have been forced into the working world of waitressing by necessity. My daughter now spends most of her time in day care, and when I really want to take a break and go out with my friends, I have to go home and be mom. As you can imagine, there aren't many guys my age who are willing to stick around long term to raise a kid. So when I actually find a guy, the relationships are short, but not very sweet. I don't regret having her, but I do regret the change in my lifestyle. I don't feel like a normal 20 year old. I am struggling to make ends meet and working all the time, while all of my friends are out partying and having fun.

This leads me to my current need to write every girl who is out there banging her head against the wall, wondering what to do about this next unplanned pregnancy. This is my second one; you would think I would have learned the first time, but apparently not. This leaves me three options, parenting is out; I can't support another child all by myself. And I don't believe in abortion, so unless I win the lottery, that leaves adoption as my best option.

At first I was having a hard time thinking how I could carry this baby for nine months and then give it to someone else. But I know I can't provide this child the life I would like them to have. I have been spending a lot of time talking with families, and there are so many that want to have a child to call their own. So far I haven't been very good at making the right decision, so maybe it's important that I think about someone other than myself. I know this is going to be a hard decision, but it is the one thing I can do to make my life and the baby's life a little better.

Jamie

Celebrities touched by adoption

Adoptive Parents

Tom Cruise & Nicole Kidman – *Actors*
Madonna – *Musician*
Calista Flockhart – *Actress*
Angelina Jolie & Brad Pitt – *Actors*
John McCain – *Politician*
Jamie Lee Curtis – *Author/Actress*
Michelle Pfieffer – *Actress*
George Lucas – *Film Producer, Star Wars*
Sheryl Crow – *Singer*
Ben Stein – *Actor and Game Show Host*
Dan Marino – *Football Player*
Diane Keaton – *Actress*
Kirk Cameron – *Actor*
Magic Johnson – *Basketball Player*
Meg Ryan – *Actress*
Ronald Reagan – *Former President*
Steven Spielberg – *Film Director*
Walt Disney – *Founder of Disney*

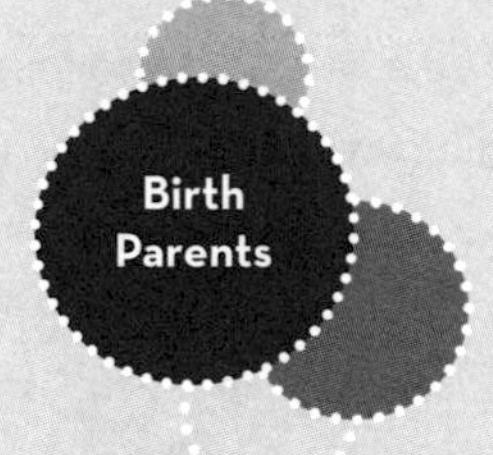

Albert Einstein – *Physicist*
Joni Mitchell – *Singer/Actress*
Rosanne Barr – *Entertainer/Actress*
Hank Williams – *Country Singer*
Kate Mulgrew – *Actress*
Mercedes Ruehl – *Actress*
Strom Thurmond – *Politician*

Adoptees

Faith Hill - *Singer*
Melissa Gilbert - *Actress, "Little House on the Prairie"*
Nicole Richie - *Actress*
Steve Jobs - *Founder of Apple Computer*
Eleanor Roosevelt - *First Lady*
Darryl McDaniels - *Rapper, Run DMC*
Jesse Jackson - *Minister/Politician*
Bill Clinton - *Former President*
John Lennon - *Musician*
Malcolm X - *Civil Rights Leader*
Nat King Cole - *Singer*
Priscilla Presley - *Actress*
Sarah McLachlan - *Singer*
Tim McGraw - *Country Singer*

Three out of five people are touched by adoption. Adoption is a decision that changes lives forever, but it can be one of the most amazing ways to bring people together. It has been a way for mothers to find peace knowing that a loving family will provide for their child.

With open adoption birth mothers and adoptive families alike can be just as involved in creating the best life for the child.

My Journal

CHAPTER SIX:

The steps to adoption...

Remember, many services are available to women making an adoption plan. Your adoption professional can refer you to a licensed family counselor to discuss any feelings you're having, at no cost to you. You can also receive help locating a doctor in your community, as well as legal and public aid. There are even educational scholarships available so you can continue your education. Call the National Adoption Hotline at 1-800-923-6602 for more information about these resources. So what do you need to do to make an adoption plan? Here are the steps to follow:

1. Request information about adoption

When you first contact an adoption professional, you will be asked a few questions. Then you can receive a packet with family profiles and a questionnaire. You can also access a great deal of information from the websites listed in the back of this book.

2. Determine your due date

Pregnancies last about 40 weeks. To find out your due date, you can use an online pregnancy due date calculator here: **www.PregnancyHelpOnline.com**. Your adoption professional can also help you calculate when you are due.

It is normal to deliver two weeks before or after your due date. You will have an ultrasound where a picture of the baby is taken using sound waves and a computer. This helps confirm the due date, the gender of the baby, and can determine if there are complications.

3. Get the assistance you need

Financial and housing help are available to you if you need it. In most states, adoptive parents can pay some of your expenses once you are matched. The adoptive parents will have an attorney who will assist them in determining what they can and can't pay for.

Dear Mardie:
"What is my baby doing at two months along?"

Mardie's Advice:
Her heart is beating, and she can turn her head, suck her thumb and respond to pain.

It is important that you are comfortable with the adoptive parents and the adoption plan you have chosen before accepting any financial assistance.

If you need help now, visit **www.BirthmotherBlessings.com** for free help with maternity clothes, household items, and other necessities.

4. Fill out the paperwork

You will be sent some basic paperwork by e-mail, regular mail, or Federal Express that you will need to fill out. This paperwork will include questions about you, your medical history, the desired level of contact you wish to have after the adoption, and a list of resources. If you have any questions or need help filling it out, just call the National Adoption Hotline at 1-800-923-6602. Once you send or fax back paperwork and a proof of your pregnancy (or a birth certificate if the child's been born), you can begin to speak with adoptive families.

5. View and select the adoptive families

You will be able to view adoptive family profiles online at the websites listed in the resources section in the back of this book. The families on these sites have been prescreened and are ready to take on the responsibilities of adoption and parenting. Your

Dear Mardie:
"No one will accept my choice. No one cares about my news. Where can I turn?"

Mardie's Advice:
Making an adoption plan is a very personal and individual decision. Some women want to share their plans with friends. Other women are more private and let no one know. You may not have anyone to speak to. If that is the case, please call Lifetime Adoption at any time day or night at 1-800-923-6784.

adoption professional will also send you longer versions of the profiles in the mail. Some women will receive a large number of profiles in the mail and others just a few. It all depends on your needs. There are families for all children regardless of age, race, or medical condition.

A good idea is to select your 1st, 2nd, and 3rd choices in adoptive parents. Don't just look at the photos, as many people may not photograph well but may be perfect for your child and you.

Each adoptive family will have a toll-free number and e-mail address to make it easy for you to contact them. Your adoption professional will call the family you are interested in to arrange a time to speak or meet them.

Here are some things to consider as you evaluate your choice of families:

- *Do you want your child raised in a particular state or area?*
- *How important is it for them to grow up with a brother or sister?*
- *What faith do you want them to be brought up with? Is this important to you?*
- *Do you think that you would like them to be in the city or country? Near mountains or the ocean?*
- *How important is it to be active in sports or outdoor activities?*
- *Are the arts important, possibly a family that enjoys classical music, ballet, opera, museums, and attending cultural events?*
- *Are pets important?*
- *Extended family, grandparents?*

6. Speak with potential families

You have the opportunity to speak with one or more potential adoptive families. If you feel uncomfortable or nervous talking with the family by yourself, your adoption professional can join you in a phone conference. This can help break the ice and ensure that your questions can be answered without putting you on the spot.

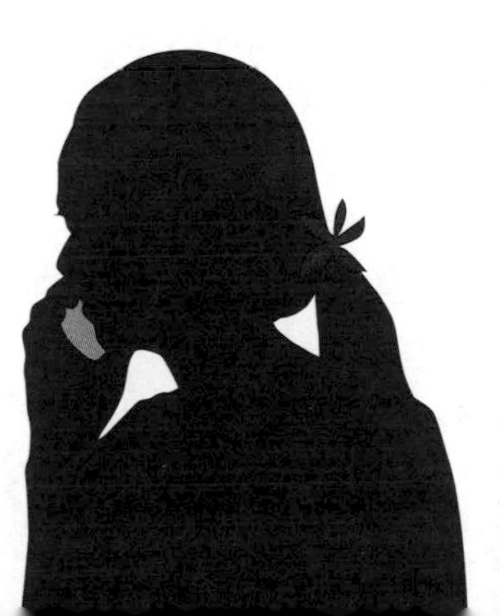

After speaking to the family, you may have an idea if they are what you are seeking for your child. If not, you are free to speak with more families. Your coordinator will be happy to arrange this for you.

Here is a list of possible questions you may wish to ask the family:

1) *Why are you adopting?*
2) *Do you have any other children? Were they adopted?*
3) *What are the other children's ages, talents, and interests?*
4) *What do you do for a living and are you financially able to provide for a child?*
5) *Do you both work? Who will care for the child when you are not with him or her?*
6) *How do you envision your adopted child's future? Hopes and dreams?*
7) *How do you plan to discipline? Spankings, time-outs, or reward systems?*
8) *What are your hobbies and family activities?*
9) *Do you attend church regularly? What religion are you, and how do you practice your faith?*
10) *What kind of involvement do you hope to have with me during the adoption process and after we finalize? Are you open to exchanging letters, photos, and having occasional visits?*

If you are uncomfortable with the adoptive parents' questions or feel they aren't treating you with respect, let them know. You are

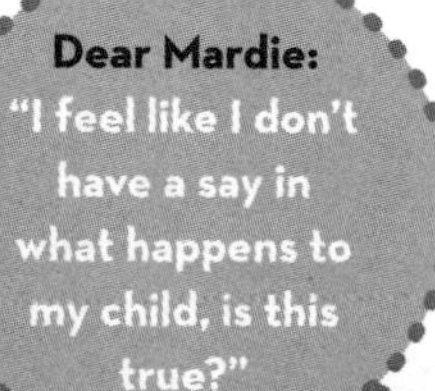

Mardie's Advice:
You have the right to be involved in all phases of the adoption process.

You have the right to:

...have answers to all of your questions, and develop a relationship with the adoptive family.

...see, hold, and spend time with the baby at birth.

...talk, meet and choose the adoptive family.

...be treated with dignity and respect for your loving decision.

...have contact, including letters, photos and visits, if you want.

not obligated to speak with them further if you don't want to.

If you are in need of financial assistance for pregnancy related expenses, please be sure to discuss this with your adoption professional as these issues need to be handled by the attorney working on your adoption. It may seem awkward to discuss financial matters with the adoptive family so leave this to your adoption coordinator.

Above all, keep in mind that no matter whom you choose it is your child's best interest that should always come first.

You can start your adoption anytime. When you are ready, you may talk with the family (or families) of your choice. Even if you call from the hospital in labor or you are a parent of an older child, you will have the opportunity to get to know the family and build a relationship.

7. A match is made

You will be considered "matched" with the adoptive parents once you have spoken with them, and both parties feel comfortable moving forward together.

If at any time you sense that the adoptive family is not such a good fit, please let your adoption professional know right away. Open communication is vital to the success of your adoption. Making sure that your needs and the needs of your child are being met is just one part of the adoption professional's role.

When you are matched with an adoptive family, you legally have no obligation. Just be sure to leave yourself enough time to find another family if you decide that this one isn't right for you. If you are struggling with your decision, turn to your adoption professional for support and advice.

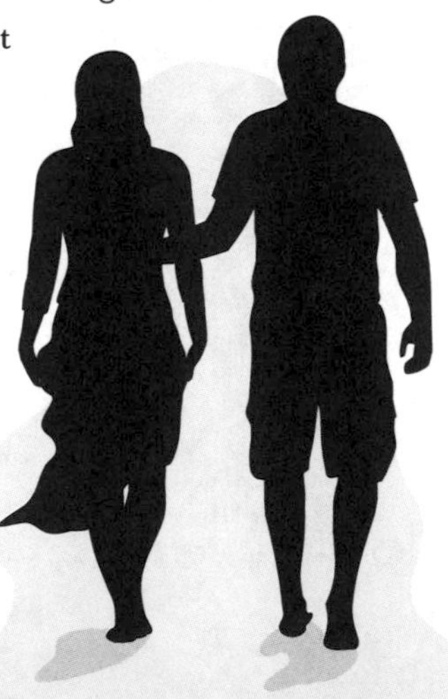

It is important that you stay in touch with your adoption professional by calling or emailing every one to two weeks or more often. Your adoption professional will put you in contact with the resources that you need during the adoption process, including professional counseling and peer counseling if you desire. You will also be connected with an adoption attorney to discuss any legal questions.

You and the adoptive family will continue to build your relationship throughout your pregnancy. It is a good time to learn about each other, and share with each other. You can discuss your hospital plan and other plans as you continue through your pregnancy.

8. Plan for delivery

Be sure to call your adoption professional and the adoptive family when you go into labor. If you would prefer, your adoption professional can call the family for you. In most cases the baby will be discharged from the hospital to the adoptive family about the same time you are released.

Be sure to call with any questions or concerns, there is someone who is available 24 hours a day, seven days a week at 1-800-923-6602. For more information on planning for delivery, see chapter 8.

Concern about Child Protective Services

If CPS or drug use has been a concern, consider giving your child the gift of a lifetime. Get private, confidential, non-judgmental answers to your questions by calling 1-800-923-6602, available 24 hours a day, seven days a week.

There is an alternative to CPS and Foster Care for your child. You may make the choice of the adoptive family for your newborn or older children. You are able to receive letters and photographs and, if desired, contact with your child.

Call before your choices are no longer yours to make. Be aware that you need to stay in contact with your adoption professional to assure that CPS does not become involved, if this is a concern of yours.

If you have used drugs or have a concern that you or your baby may test positive for drugs at delivery, you can still make an adoption plan; call 1-800-923-6602, 24 hours a day, seven days a week.

9. Sign legal documents

You will meet with an attorney or adoption service provider who will advise you of your rights and help you review the legal documents required to complete this part of the adoption. This may be done in the hospital or a different location after you have been discharged.

10. Heal

You will need to take time to heal your body and your heart. Give yourself time; plan for this. Be patient. For more information on giving yourself time to heal, see chapter 9.

CHAPTER SEVEN:

Taking care of you...

With so much going on, the emotional changes, thoughts about your future, as well as the baby's future, it can be hard to deal with the day to day. It is important to be aware of your needs and to take the time to make healthy choices. This can help you feel better emotionally and physically during the duration of your pregnancy.

Doctor's appointments

Try to keep all your doctor's appointments. Even if you have had a child before, it is good to receive the care you need to during this pregnancy. If you have trouble getting there, let your adoption professional or adoptive family know. Doctor's appointments are important to you and your baby's health. If you would like, ask the adoptive mother to come with you to your appointments. The adoptive father may come as well, if you are comfortable with this, or he can stay in the waiting room. Having the adoptive family at the appointments can be a great time to get to know them. They can be a wonderful source of support.

The family will appreciate the chance to know how you are feeling, as well as the health of the baby. When you have your ultrasounds, you may want to share copies with the adoptive family. Sharing updates from your doctor's appointments is a great way to keep them involved and supportive of your health.

First visit to the doctor or medical clinic

Your first visit may be longer than others, so plan some time. You may feel more comfortable if you bring someone who cares along on this first visit. If you have little ones, bring someone to watch them in the waiting room while you are being examined. There may be a lot of paperwork to be completed.

The doctor will need to know about your adoption plan. Once you know the name of the doctor or clinic that will be caring for you, let your adoption professional know. She will handle the paperwork to obtain the medical records she needs regarding your pregnancy.

In most cases, you will be asked to return to the doctor every four weeks for the first seven months.

Then, every two weeks until the last month, then every week. If problems arise, you may be scheduled for more frequent visits.

During the pregnancy, there should be an exchange of ideas. Consider what your doctor suggests and why. It's important that you share your hospital preferences with your doctor once you get closer to your due date. Your adoption professional will fax a copy of your hospital preference to that hospital. Remember that your doctor has experience that can be valuable to you during pregnancy and beyond.

Mental health

Try to keep an eye on your mental health and your emotions. You may feel weepy during your pregnancy. If you start to feel unusually depressed, let your doctor, adoption professional or adoptive parents know at once. Here are some signs of depression:

- *Inability to sleep due to anxiety*
- *Inability to find enjoyment in your life*
- *Feelings of sadness or anxiety that last longer than two weeks*
- *Eating too much or too little*
- *Obsessive thoughts that won't go away*
- *Thoughts of suicide*

Some of these thoughts are normal at any time. However, when they begin to get in the way of your normal daily life, it is time to seek help. Your adoption professional is there to help you. Call her.

Weight and pregnancy

Don't try to lose weight during your pregnancy; it will hurt both you and the baby. Your doctor will give you guidelines on the normal amount of weight to gain, based on your height and on your weight before you became pregnant.

The baby is going to use nutrients from you and if you don't replenish your body you will suffer. If you are having trouble getting the proper foods, please let your adoption professional know about it immediately.

Tips for overcoming nausea

If you are suffering from nausea, try to eat smaller meals throughout the day. Quite often, when you get up in the morning, your tummy will be full of acid. A little bread or a saltine cracker can do the trick by soaking up any acid left over from the night before; also ginger ale and carbonated beverages can help. SEA Bands™ are cloth bands that are worn on your wrists and can help reduce nausea. These bands can be found in drug stores. If you can't afford them or can't find them, let your adoption professional or adoptive parents know and they can send you some. Your doctor may have additional tips on how to manage nausea during pregnancy.

Drug and alcohol use

You may have used drugs or alcohol before you knew you were pregnant or you may be continuing to use. It is important for your health and the health of the baby to be honest about the type of drug use and the frequency of use so that your physician can take care of your needs appropriately. There can be long term health effects, such as the possibility of lower birth weight if there is continued tobacco use.

Although it may seem tempting to conceal any drug or alcohol use, it is very helpful for both the adoptive professional and the adoptive families to know everything upfront. Whatever situation you find yourself in, there are lots of wonderful families who are more than willing to adopt a child that may have drug or alcohol exposure.

Please be aware that if you are actively using drugs close to your delivery date, your baby may test positive. If your child tests positive for drug exposure, hospital staff is *required* to notify Child Protective Services. There is a strong chance that the child will be removed from your care and put into foster care, unless you make an adoption plan. You *always* have the right to make an adoption plan.

Finding prenatal care

You may already have a doctor you prefer to see for your prenatal care (health care for you while you are pregnant). If you don't have insurance, you can apply for state-funded health insurance or emergency Medicaid, allowing you to see a doctor right away.

You can find OB-GYN doctors (physicians specializing in female reproductive systems) in your area by checking the yellow pages in your local phone book or by searching the internet. Here are some possible keywords to use in your search: "doctors," "physicians," "women's health care," "obstetrics," and "gynecology" along with the city and state you live in. Search for local hospitals and doctors by going to **www.BigYellow.com** and typing in your state and city.

Caring for yourself

The first three months of pregnancy are the most important time for you to take care of yourself. Getting the proper medical care and diet can make all the difference in the world. Prenatal vitamins and a balanced diet can keep your emotions balanced and your body strong. Try to avoid caffeine, raw seafood, unpasteurized milk, soft cheeses (as they contain bacteria that can harm your baby), and herbs or herbal tea (unless OK'd by your doctor).

If you do not have medical insurance, be sure to tell your adoption professional. She can arrange to find the care you need, in a medical center or hospital that is near you.

Questions for my doctor

My doctor: ______________________ Phone number: ______________________

My hospital: ______________________ Phone number: ______________________

CHAPTER EIGHT

Planning for delivery...

Planning your adoption day

Getting ready for the delivery can be a nervous and anxious time. It can help to prepare a little ahead of time, so that you have less to think about when your contractions start.

Many women who are choosing adoption for their child feel uneasy packing their hospital bag. **BirthmotherBlessings.com** will send you a FREE hospital bag with some of the necessities. Call 1-800-923-6602 and ask for a free labor bag.

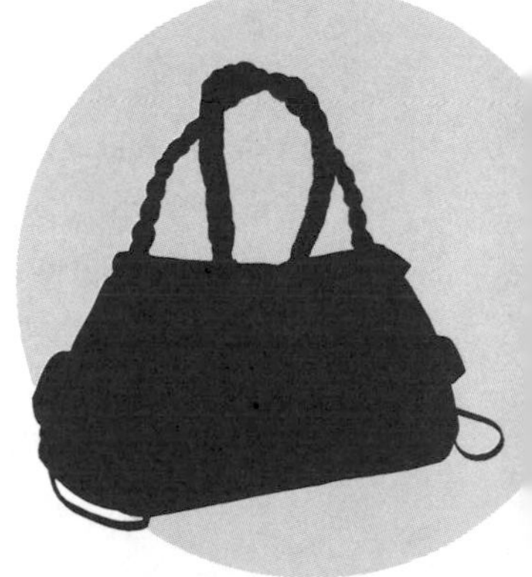

Here is a list of things you can do in advance of your adoption day:

1) *Tour the labor and delivery area of the hospital and ask about pre-registering at the hospital.*
2) *Plan to take time off work. You may be eligible for pregnancy disability leave both before and after the birth. Check with your physician and your employer for the proper documents.*
3) *Sign up for childbirth classes, if you feel this knowledge would be helpful to you.*
4) *Decide on your hospital preferences and write them down. Make copies and send one to your adoption professional, this ensures your wishes are known.*
5) *Decide who you want to be at the hospital with you when you deliver. If you have other children, arrange for someone to take care of them while you are in the hospital.*
6) *Have your bag packed and ready to go.*
7) *Decide who will pick you up from the hospital when you are discharged.*
8) *Do you want the baby in the room with you, or would you prefer the baby be kept in the nursery with the adoptive parents?*
9) *Do you want to be in a different area of the hospital away from the labor and delivery area?*
10) *How much do you want the adoptive parents to participate in the birth? Do you want them in the delivery room or waiting outside?*
11) *If you want newborn pictures, let the hospital know.*
12) *When you are discharged, do you want to wait until the baby leaves or do you wish to leave first?*

What do I do when I go into labor?

Let your adoption professional know when your labor starts and when you leave for the hospital or when you get there. Your adoption professional will send paperwork to the hospital staff to ensure they have your hospital preferences and desires available and your wishes are followed. Give the labor nurse your adoption professional's phone number and ask her to call them. Your adoption professional can notify the adoptive parents that you are in labor, or you may want to call them yourself.

I was shocked to find out I was pregnant... again. I had no job, my life was a mess and I didn't want another child, especially under the circumstances. I had had a one-night stand with some guy at a party. My first reaction was fear. I couldn't imagine being a single parent...again. I couldn't go through with an abortion. I decided on adoption and called an adoption center. I went through the process of choosing a family. I talked to a couple of families and I had a chance to meet the family I liked talking to. It was a great experience. They were wonderful people. I really felt for them in their struggle to have a baby. I decided that they were the ones who deserved to raise my child. They were very supportive through the rest of my pregnancy. We talked every week and became good friends too through all this. Then, when it came time for the birth, they came to my hometown. They stayed until I left the hospital three days later. It was a wonderful time! It made me happy to see the joy in their lives. I hated to see them go. We still keep in touch and I will always know how the baby is, as well as knowing he's in good hands. Now I can go on and make a better life for myself. It was a tough choice, but I know I did the right thing.

Dawn

What happens at the hospital?

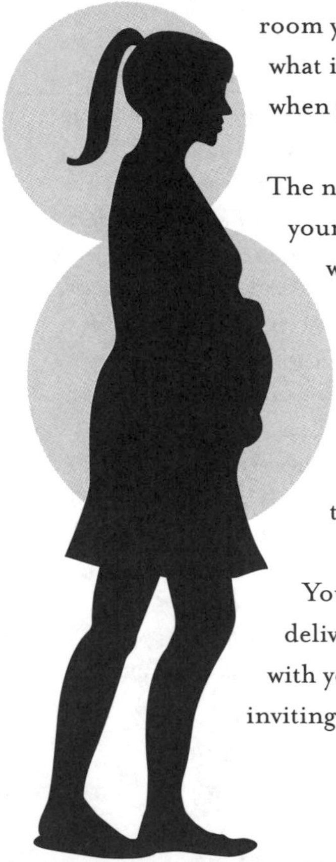

You will be taken into a labor room where your labor will be monitored. In most hospitals, this may be the same room you give birth in or you may be taken to what is traditionally called a "delivery room" when you are ready.

The nursing staff will attach a heart monitor to your tummy to make sure everything is going well with the baby. If you have attended childbirth classes, you will know what to expect during your labor. If not, the nurses are very helpful. Remember that you have rights and this is your birth and your adoption plan, so don't let anyone talk you out of what you want.

You decide who you want or don't want in the delivery room with you. Make sure the person with you is positive and well-informed before inviting them to your delivery.

Before you leave the hospital

You are encouraged to see and hold your baby. It is very healing and can help you in the grieving process. Take the time you need with your child. You can take photos; keep the baby's ID bracelet, and/or footprints.

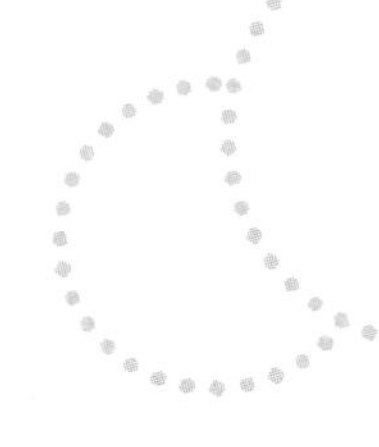

Don't leave the hospital until you are ready. If you had a C-section, you will have to stay longer to prevent infection. If you want, you can have a small ceremony to celebrate placing your child with the adoptive parents.

Did you know you can name your baby?

Naming your child allows you to create a special bond. You may want to decide with the adoptive parents, or you may want a personal name, realizing that the adoptive parents will be naming the child also. One adoptive family honored their boy's birth mother by keeping the first and middle names that his birth father had given him; they used them as their son's middle names.

Remember that all situations are different, but open, honest communication is the place to start.

Paula's Story

One day I discovered I was pregnant and facing the most difficult decision of my life. My thoughts changed overnight with the realization of the life that grew inside of me. As my pregnancy progressed, I had to decide whether or not to parent my child. As a single woman, I found the realities of parenthood to be unfair to my child. After many hours of prayer and soul-searching, I decided to make an adoption plan for my baby.

I took the time to research prospective families with Lifetime Adoption Center and found a family whom I truly loved. Together we got through my pregnancy, sharing the joys of the life that grew inside me. I had chosen my baby's adoptive mother to be my labor partner. She went to every doctor's appointment with me, and to breakfast afterward. During this time spent together, we got to know one another very well and became good friends. I felt that it was important to spend the time and effort to get to know my child's adoptive parents.

I delivered a beautiful, healthy baby girl. The time spent in the hospital was almost magical; together with my daughter's parents, I was able to care for her. We spent 36 hours in the hospital sharing with friends and family the beautiful life that I had created. It was a time of love and laughter. Emotions ran high in those few hours, but the one that was most present was LOVE!

After we parted and went home, I with my family and my daughter with hers, I knew that my daughter was loved and cared for in a way that only a two parent family can provide. I love my daughter with all my heart, and because of that love I was able to give her everything I had always wanted for her. I know that open adoption was the very best option for my daughter, Alexandra.

Today I am able to share my story with others with the hope of educating as many people as possible about the benefits of open adoption. As a birth mother, I will never have to hide behind a veil of secrecy, and I will always know how my daughter is doing. I do wish I had been in a position to parent her myself, but I am so very excited for the life she will be able to lead due to open adoption. Each and every day I think of my daughter and know that she is loved, safe, and thriving in her home.

I can see from the photos and letters that the adoptive parents regularly send me that she is growing into a lovely young girl. The relationship that my daughter's adoptive parents and I share is one that will last a lifetime.

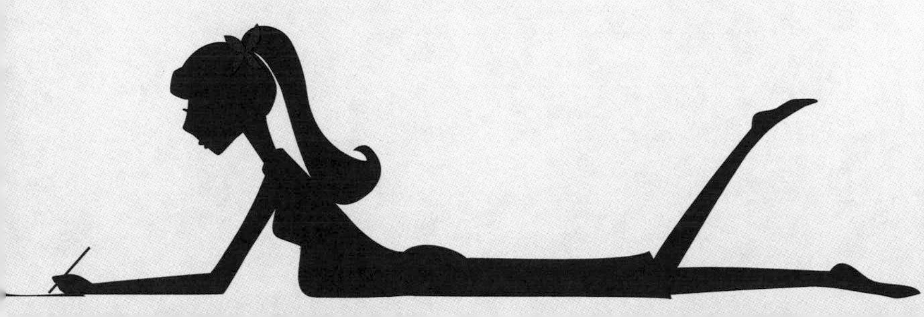

My hospital checklist

- ☐ *Coordinator's number*
- ☐ *Adoptive family's number*
- ☐ *Labor bag*
- ☐ *Purse*
- ☐ *Insurance/Medicaid card*
- ☐ ______________________
- ☐ ______________________
- ☐ ______________________
- ☐ ______________________
- ☐ ______________________
- ☐ ______________________
- ☐ ______________________
- ☐ ______________________
- ☐ ______________________
- ☐ ______________________

CHAPTER NINE:

Getting by & moving on...

Before, during, and after your adoption, take time for yourself. Deciding to place your child in an adoption plan is a life-changing event for you. Don't be hard on yourself; it is not realistic to expect everything to go back to the way it used to be. You will change from this experience. Acknowledging that this is the right decision for you is the first thing you can do to help yourself. After delivery, you are still in the post-pregnancy hormone adjustment stage. It is difficult to look at anything with much clarity, but it will get better. Concentrate on letting your body heal itself from pregnancy and birth.

Your feelings

Remember that just because you feel sadness, it doesn't mean your decision was wrong. Sometimes you will have delayed grief that may not surface for a few weeks or months. When those times

??

Dear Mardie:
"I still have weight to lose from my pregnancy and this makes me think of my baby. Is this normal?"

Mardie's Advice:
Be patient with yourself as you heal from labor and adjust to life after pregnancy. It is normal to feel sad and reflective. Some women find that it helps to focus on the future. You want to avoid stuffing your feelings inside. Let your feelings be felt and then focus on the reasons you personally had for the adoption. Speaking to other women who have gone through adoption can help. You will not forget your child, but with time the feelings will become less intense, and you may even find them comforting. Call your adoption professional if you would like to speak to another birth mother or a counselor.

come, seek help from professionals or other birth mothers. Call your adoption professional. Often, she can offer you mentoring or provide you with the name of a counselor in your area. Some counselors even offer to do over-the-phone counseling with birth mothers in crisis. Call your physician, as they will have counseling referrals as well.

The Internet is filled with forums and chat rooms where you can share your emotions. You will learn how to place one foot in front of the other and make it through to the next day. You will also learn that it is possible to live again. You will laugh and you will find comfort in knowing that what you did was the greatest thing of all. You have given *life* a chance.

What can you do today?

Build up a group of people who support your decision. Try to offset negative people with at least two positive people in your life. If possible, stay clear of negative influences until you are stronger.

You can make positive changes in your life by going back to school, church, or getting a new job. Make new friends and try new places.

Staying away from anything that would lead back to an old habit could be helpful. If you know you have a weakness, like drugs, alcohol, or being attracted to the wrong guys, seek help from a counselor trained in that area. Try to prevent yourself from getting hurt while you are in a vulnerable place.

If you have a history of depression or bi-polar disorder, your symptoms may worsen so seek help at your earliest opportunity. Stay on your medication and be sure to see your doctor.

As time passes, the pain and sadness will fade. You won't ever forget your child, but it does get better. Whenever we lose something or have to let go of someone, we feel some level of grief and your heart will be heavy for some time. It is normal to feel grief for a while after the adoption.

You can take pride in having given your child life and the best possible environment in which to live and grow.

Ongoing contact

After you have been discharged from the hospital and your baby is with his or her adoptive parents, you will begin the healing process, moving forward to reach your own goals. You may need to meet with a social worker or your attorney to sign additional papers.

"If I hadn't chosen adoption, I wouldn't have seen the joy it brought to the couple that couldn't have children.

- Lisa in Kansas

You may wish to consider what kind of contact you want with your child after the adoption. Do you want to have an ongoing relationship with your child and his or her adoptive parents? Some women choose to send their photos to their adoption professional, who then forwards them on to the adoptive parents. The adoptive family can post their pictures on the Internet for you to view as often as you like. You can also have contact by e-mail or regular mail if you prefer.

The type of contact you want with your child and the adoptive family may change over time. It is important to be honest with yourself and the adoptive family so that everyone can be open and communicate about what is in the best interest of the child.

Your future, goals, and dreams

Your future is up to you. Now is the time to use the lessons you have learned. What do you want to do with your life? You have *given* the greatest gift in the world. Now it is time to give *yourself* the greatest gift - a future with a plan. It's okay for you to dream of a better future and to dream of a better life. Where do you want to go and what do you want to do?

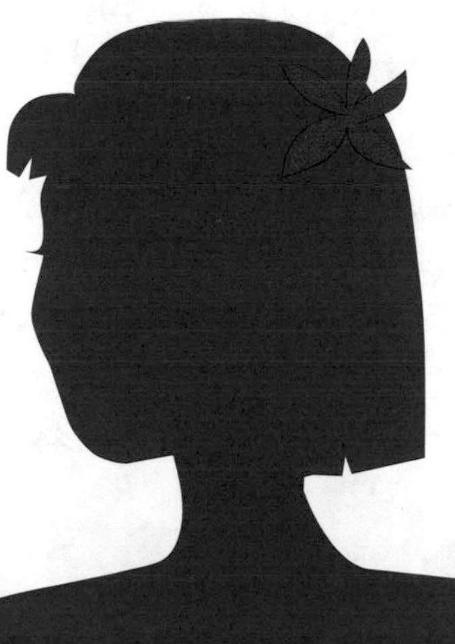

Dear Mardie: *"I keep hearing throughout my pregnancy that I should plan for my future after the adoption, is this selfish?"*

Mardie's Advice: *Looking forward and into your future can help you focus on the reason for your adoption. Remember you are not a bad person for doing so.*

Timing is everything and at this time in your life, parenting a child may not be possible. This is a loving and selfless decision women make for their children. Instead of parenting a child, they realize they are not in a position to offer them what they need at this time in their lives.

Dear Mardie: *"I seem to think of my child often. Is it normal to feel sad sometimes?"*

Mardie's Advice: *You may find yourself remembering your child and what could have been. This is normal. Let the memories come, talk about your feelings and when possible, journal your thoughts. These emotions are part of the post-adoption process, sadness might come and go- it doesn't stop just because the pregnancy is over. In fact, you might find your emotions building up each year on or around your child's birthday or placement date. This is very normal.*

Dear Mardie: *"Is it ok to go out with friends and have fun, I feel so guilty?"*

Mardie's Advice: *Having some fun and getting back into life does not mean you don't love your child. It is not a betrayal. Giving yourself permission to have some fun and happiness is good for you and your healing, just like you must give yourself permission to grieve when you have the need.*

Dear Mardie: *"My friends and family are always trying to cheer me up. Sometimes they don't even know how to respond to me. What can I do to let them know how I feel?"*

Mardie's Advice: *You may want to share some boundaries with concerned friends who are determined not to let you be sad or alone. Remember, they may not be sure how to handle your feelings. Let others know what you need and how they can best help you. Don't feel pressured into doing things you don't want to do or don't feel up to – just to keep others happy. Decide what and how much you need, and then share these feelings with others.*

"I know I can obtain a positive place in the world. I also know that by continuing my education, I can set an example for other girls in my situation -that you can do anything you put your mind to. I know my child will be proud."

- Jessica,a birthmother receiving a Lifetime Foundation scholarship

Working on the future

It is helpful if you can try to take little steps toward your future. If you haven't finished high school, making one phone call can help you work toward your high school diploma. Tomorrow you can take another little step, such as making an appointment at your school's office or finding out how to study for the GED test.

If you plan to get a job, it is useful for you to start by making a list of your talents and abilities. The next day, you might look at a few examples of resumes. This will help you to see how you should create your own resume. Once you have created a resume, you can make an appointment with an employment agency, which will help you on your job hunt. By doing one small thing each day, you will move closer to achieving your future goals.

Educational scholarship

Did you know there is a scholarship program developed solely for women who have lovingly chosen adoption for their children? Lifetime Foundation is dedicated to the development of healthy and fulfilling futures. All children need a loving family who can provide guidance, opportunity, and the promise of a full life. Birth mothers deserve the opportunity for a positive future after adoption in the same way they have ensured a healthy future for their child. For an application and for more information, please visit: **www.LifetimeAdoptionFoundation.org.**

Emotional changes

You are going to have some worries, so it is a good idea to share them with your adoption professional and those close to you. If you have no close family or friends, there are other people ready to help you. Sometimes it is easier to share your concerns with an outside person such as the adoption social worker, counselor, or pastor. If you are not sure how to find these people, just ask your adoption professional for referrals.

The fear and worry you might have felt during your pregnancy, and the loss and sadness you feel about your baby can get in the way of a relationship. It's not unusual for you to fear that an unplanned pregnancy could happen again. This is a normal reaction, but it is not a healthy way to live your life. Be very honest about how you are feeling about sex and intimacy. You might ask your boyfriend or husband to join you after your first meeting with the counselor. This should help him understand how you feel. Your counselor can help the two of you work this problem out together.

My Journal

My Journal

My Journal

CHAPTER TEN:

My adoption choice...

Placing your child for adoption is a personal choice, one that takes time and consideration to make. Ask lots of questions and talk to an adoption professional. Know what options are available to you and then take your time to decide.

Your feelings and concerns are yours, but you are not alone with these feelings, they are a normal piece to the larger adoption process. Whether you are just making your decisions now or have completed the adoption of your child, know that you are in good company with thousands of women who have chosen adoption for their child.

Adoption professionals have worked with women from all backgrounds, in many different situations and have compassionate answers to your questions. Take the time to explore your options and come to the best decision for you and your child.

This journey takes courage and strength, but you have taken the first step just by choosing to pick up this book. Knowing your options can bring you peace and encouragement as you continue on your journey.

Dear Mardie:

The last few months have been the hardest stretch in my life. The choices & decisions that I've been faced with will be with me forever. From the beginning you and my adoption coordinator have been there for me, I could not have done this without all of you and your love and support. You will forever by my Lifetime family. I know that I made the right choice for me and my child!

~Lizzy

Once you have made your decision, you can map out your choices for an adoptive family, your adoption plan and your future goals. Know that your adoption professional is available to help you anytime.

For more information or to speak to someone about your options, please call 1-800-923-6602; there is someone on staff 24 hours a day, 7 days a week.

Recipe for Adoption Success

2 cups of conversation, it's good to talk about your feelings.
1 cup of listening to what your inner voice is saying.
3 cups of honesty, be honest with yourself.
½ cup of reality, be clear with your expectations of yourself.
1 tsp. of help, don't be afraid to ask for counseling.
1¼ cup of feelings, yours not your parents or friends.
1 cup journaling, writing down your thoughts.
1 cup of planning, your adoption, your choices.
3 cups understanding, that you will have good days and bad.
3 tsp. each of long term goals and **support**,
a pinch of grief, it's normal.
Adoptive Parents, hand picked.
A Lifetime of Pride, in yourself and your decision.

Mix together conversation, honesty, help and listening. Fold in reality and support.

In a separate bowl mix planning, feelings, journaling, understanding, and grief. Combine the two. Add the long term goals and pride. Pour mixture into baking dish, season for 9 months. Top with love for your child.

The recipe will result in a beautiful gift of success and love, knowing that you have created a wonderful life for your child.

My Choices

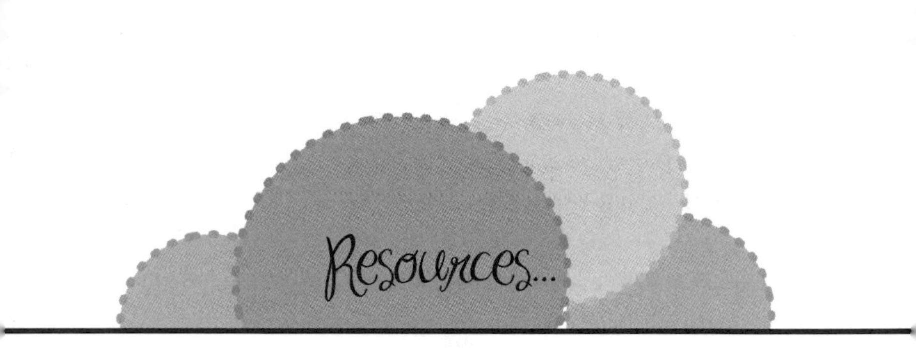

Online Adoption Resources

- **NationalAdoptionHotline.com** 1-800-923-6602
  Staffed 24/7, call today.
- **www.LifetimeAdoption.com** 1-800-9-ADOPT-4
  Nationwide adoption center providing free services, maternity clothes, housing assistance, and more. Available twenty-four hours a day.
- **www.OpenAdoption.com**
  Choose the family and a very open relationship.
- **AfricanAmericanAdoptionsOnline.com**
  Pre-approved families eagerly waiting to adopt African American and mixed race children.
- **www.Biracial-Adoptions.com**
  View waiting families seeking biracial children.

- **CatholicAdoptionOnline.com**
  #1 place for finding waiting Catholic families.
- **www.HispanicAdoptionServices.com**
  Specializing in adoption for Hispanic families.
- **UnplannedPregnancy.blogspot.com**
  Blog for women facing an unplanned pregnancy.
- **ChristianAdoptionHotline.com**
  Nonjudgmental help and advice 24 hours a day.

Additional Resources

- **www.LifetimeFoundation.org** 530-432-7383
  Providing Birthmother Educational Scholarships and other assistance to women choosing adoption.
- **www.PregnancyHelpOnline.com**
  Pregnancy options, articles and more! Live chat!
- **www.16andPregnant.com**
  Many teens have been where you are. There is hope after unplanned pregnancy.
- **www.StatebyStateAdoptions.com**
  Choose a family waiting to adopt in your state.
- **www.BirthMotherCounseling.com**
  Sometimes you just need someone to talk to.

Glossary of Adoption Terms

Adoptee: *A child who is adopted and joins a family through adoption.*

Adoption Attorney: *A lawyer who specializes in adoption and knows the process completely. Paid for by the adoptive family.*

Adoption Facilitator: *An organization who brings together birth families and adoptive parents, assisting in building an adoption plan. Facilitators specialize in meeting the needs of the people in the adoption plan.*

Adoption Plan: *An individual plan made by the birth mother for the adoption of her child. Includes the type of family she wishes to adopt her child, who will be at the birth and the amount of contact between the adoptive parents, adoptee, and birth parents following the adoption.*

Adoption Service Provider (ASP): *A licensed social worker who is certified by the state to assist with the placement of a child.*

Adoption Triad: *The three parties involved in an adoption; birth parents, adoptive parents, and adopted child/children.*

Adoptive Parent: *A person who becomes the permanent parent through adoption with all the legal rights and moral responsibilities given to any parent.*

Birth Father: *The biological father.*

Birth Mother: *The biological mother.*

Birth Parent: *Parents who gave birth to a child, made an adoption plan for, and placed that child for adoption.*

Closed Adoption: *An adoption in near total confidentiality with no contact or ongoing relationship.*

Confidentiality: *All information kept private and not disclosed.*

Consent: *Agreement by a parent to relinquish the child for adoption and to release all rights and duties with respect to that child.*

Decree of Adoption: *A legal order that finalizes an adoption.*

Father's Adoption Registry: *Created for birth fathers in a few states who want to receive notice if plans are made to place his child for adoption.*

Foster Care: *An arrangement through a social services agency or court in which someone other than the birth parents care for the child.*

Guardian: *Person who is legally responsible for the care of a child.*

Independent Adoption: *An adoption handled by facilitators/agencies and attorneys.*

Maternity Home: *A home for unmarried pregnant women needing housing.*

Open Adoption: *Allows the birth mother to have choices about the family that adopts her child, meetings before and/or after the child's birth, ability of adoptive parents to attend the birth, continued relationship between families through letters, photos, videos, or personal visits.*

Paternity Testing: *Genetic tests that prove or disprove the identity of a child's alleged father.*

Profile: *A packet that provides information about prospective adoptive parents, usually including photos and letters. Some profiles share more about extended family, religion, lifestyle, home, and hobbies that assist the birth mother in making a choice in adoptive families.*

Putative Father: *Legal term for the alleged or believed father of a child.*

Relinquishment: *Voluntary termination of parental rights, releasing the child for adoption.*

Semi-open Adoption: *An adoption in which some information is shared, but more limited than a fully open adoption.*

Special Needs Adoption: *Older children, sibling groups, children facing physical, emotional or intellectual challenges may all be considered special needs adoptions.*

My Journey

My Journey

My Journey

About the Author

Mardie Caldwell, C.O.A.P., is a nationally recognized authority on adoption. A Certified Open Adoption Practitioner, Caldwell founded Lifetime Adoption Center in 1986. Caldwell has assisted in over 1,800 successful adoptions nationwide.

Caldwell is dedicated to educating and helping birth parents and adoptive parents through teaching, speaking, writing, and her radio talk show.

Author of a number of award winning books, Caldwell has made over 150 appearances on television, including NBC's The Today Show, CNN, Fox, MSNBC, PBS, BBC, and Dr. Laura. She has been featured on numerous national radio shows and is widely sought for print articles.

Caldwell is CFO of Lifetime Adoption Foundation, a 501(c)3 non-profit charity providing grants, college scholarships, and basic necessities to birthmothers.

Order Form

Order online: AmericanCarriageHousePublishing.com

Email orders: info@CarriageHousePublishing.com

Fax orders: 1-877-423-6783

Telephone orders: 1-877-423-6785

Postal Orders: American Carriage House Publishing

P.O. Box 1130, Nevada City, CA 95959

Please send the following books: ______________________________

____

Name: ______________ Title: ______________

Address: ______________ City: ________ State: ____ Zip: ______

Telephone: ______________ Email address: ______________

Cost per book: US $8.95

Sales tax: Please add 7.375% for products shipped to California addresses.

Shipping: US $4.50 for first book, $2.25 for each additional copy

International $9.95 for first book, $4.95 for each additional

(shipping may vary depending on destination)

Payment: ❑ Check ❑ Visa ❑ MasterCard

Card Number: ______________________________

Name on card: ______________________________

Exp. date: ______________ CCV security code (3 or 4 digits): ________

Contact the publisher at 1-877-423-6785 for volume discounts.